Psychology of Childbearing

Nora Tisdall

MA, BSc(Hons), BA, SRN, RM, ADM, PGCEA

Books for Midwives Press
An imprint of Hochland & Hochland Ltd

Published by Books for Midwives Press, 174a Ashley Road, Hale, Cheshire, WA15 9SF, England.

© 1997, Nora Tisdall

First edition

ISBN 1-898507-28-7

British Library Cataloguing in Publication Data
A catalogue record for this book is available from the British Library

Printed in Great Britain by Redwood Books, Trowbridge, Wiltshire

Dedication

This work is dedicated to my late mother Mary Christine O'Hara, a remarkable woman, the mother of twelve children, and a supreme example of motherhood.

Contents

Acknowledgements

My grateful thanks to my husband Alan for his patience, advice and support.

My thanks also to my children, Katrina, Aidan, Olivia and Michael for their encouragement.

CHAPTER ONE

Introduction

Relevance of psychology

You may have wondered why psychology has become such an important topic in relation to health care in recent years. Psychology is not a new idea; it has been a recognized discipline since the 1870s. So what is psychology? The word *psychology* comes from the Greek *psyche* – the mind, soul or spirit and the word *logos* – a study or discourse. Wilhelm Wundt in 1879 was one of the first to open a laboratory in Germany for the purpose of studying the mind.

As health practitioners it is important that we have a knowledge and understanding of the theories and research which underpin our practice. Psychology, although a relatively new area of study, is in many ways the pivot on which the quality of care is assessed by both the client and by colleagues. Our awareness of psychological issues has already been increased by our experiential learning. Years of clinical practice have given practitioners some empirical knowledge of how individuals react in certain situations.

Developing this understanding and knowledge of why people react as they do can enable practitioners to care for clients in a more sensitive and empathic way. Clinical experience will show you that individuals do not always behave in an expected or socially accepted 'normal' way. A knowledge of psychology will help practitioners to understand that it is not simply that single event which has led to this displayed behaviour but a number of events in both the recent and distant past which will contribute to the response. It is well known that tears and laughter are close allies, but in some situations laughter may seem very inappropriate but nevertheless normal. To give one example, a colleague, who was already under stress because her mother was in an Intensive Care Unit and her mother-in-law was simultaneously in a Coronary Care Unit in a different hospital, was told that her brother had been involved in a road traffic accident and was in a third hospital seriously injured. She laughed in disbelief.

Her socially unacceptable reaction to the news shocked her colleagues who were unaware of the emotional context in which she received the news.

Childbearing is a stressful event, not just in labour, but throughout the pregnancy, and the stress continues through the early parenting process. Individual mothers may react in a wide variety of ways to the same stimulus and much depends on what has happened to that individual prior to the pregnancy.

Practitioners need a knowledge and understanding of how they can influence clients' attitudes to their care. As midwives, it is important for us to understand that it is not simply what is said to a client that matters, but that the way in which it is said and the social context is also very important. Our private and public (professional) selves may differ considerably in a variety of social contexts. The body language, the eye contact and facial expression, the proximity of the speaker and the significance of others in the immediate area will have an impact on the way in which information is given and received.

A client may have had a poor experience with a health professional which may adversely influence the way in which they respond to another health professional. The class and culture of the professional will be portrayed in the interaction and it may be acceptable to the client, but equally it may be that the client does not feel that they relate well to that professional. For example, the use of professional terminology can be off-putting for a client who uses a relatively limited vocabulary and hence the level of understanding may be limited. Conversely, to talk in a too simplistic way may appear patronising. Most clients will be familiar with medical terminology relating to their anatomy but may not appreciate particular details of conditions which may be obvious to a health professional.

When language which is too simple or too complex is used, it tends to increase anxiety and reduces understanding. This leads to poor communication. Communication is the key to effective care. The more a client understands of her care, the more participation she can take in the plan of care and consequently the more control she will feel she has over the decisions made regarding her care.

Application to client care

Psychology affects all areas of practice. Health care practitioners need to have an insight into their own attitudes, values and psychological state of mind because we, too, are influenced by psychological stresses in the provision of care. Attitude will be discussed in more detail in Chapter 4.

The psychological issue which has the greatest impact on the client is the issue of normality. Almost every woman (and her partner) will be anxious throughout the pregnancy, asking themselves, 'Is my baby normal'. Pregnant women dream about their babies and fantasize about their looks and behaviour. All women *expect* their baby to be normal and healthy, but care during pregnancy is focused on detecting the abnormal, whilst maintaining the normal. Consequently, even a simple test, such as assessing blood pressure, can increase a woman's anxiety. So too, does the battery of 'tests' which are carried out. Health professionals encourage all women to undergo tests to 'check that all is normal'. The implication is that if it is not normal we can and should intervene. However, it is not always possible or appropriate to intervene. That does not mean that the tests should not be carried out, but as health professionals we need to consider the relevance of all the tests on an individual client need basis.

We encourage women to participate in their care and to have some measure of control over their care through the implementation of informed consent, but the reality is that we only allow selective informed consent. On some issues, such as HIV testing, we normally engage in lengthy exchange of information. However, with the issue of the use of ultrasound, for example, very limited information is normally given, and yet ultrasound is used widely during pregnancy. It is unrealistic to expect the advantages and disadvantages of every procedure to be discussed because of the pressure of time, but equally, as professionals we have to consider what we mean by ' informed consent' and be sure that what we are practising is not in fact 'informed coercion'.

Antenatal tests can be reassuring but most expectant mothers will always be anxious to some degree about the normality of her child until she can see, hold and examine the baby in her arms after birth. Too much reassurance can cease to be reassuring and it is important to maintain a balance in the support and advice given during care.

Holistic approach to care

A holistic approach to care is not a new idea. Plato in the fourth century BC advocated that 'the cure of the part should not be attempted without treatment of the whole'. The term 'holistic' comes from the Greek *holos* meaning whole. The whole person includes the body, mind and spirit of the individual. Nowadays that could be considered to be the physical being, the psychological being and the sociocultural being. Care cannot consider only one element, but needs to consider the context of wellbeing and the influences on the individual who is undergoing a form of stress. The individual's response to any event or condition will be affected by all aspects of his or her person. Consequently, a supportive and empathic carer and environment, together with the element of control of one's destiny will improve the outcome not exacerbate the condition.

With increasing specialization in the field of health care, professionals have honed their area of study. This has tended to blinker the professional to the wider issues of personal wellbeing – that of psychological and sociocultural wellbeing. Psychological care is as important to maintaining the feeling of satisfaction with care as is the physical aspect of care. If the anxieties and concerns of clients are not expressed, or are not *actively* listened to by carers, then the feeling of being cared for is minimized. Psychological care needs to be an implicit part of holistic care, together with consideration of the sociocultural background from which the client comes, the norms and values of which will influence the decisions made regarding care, particularly the sociocultural practices surrounding childbearing.

Psychological care is fundamental to good care during childbearing. Childbearing is a stressful life event and Niven (1994) argues that 'becoming a parent is stressful'. Anxieties regarding the pregnancy and labour are a persistent concern to women, their partners and their wider family. In addressing the psychological needs of women and their families in the approach to care the health professional endeavours to meet the needs and wants of the whole person for whom she is caring and in doing so improves the perceived quality of care. Childbearing is not a state of ill-health but of an altered state of health which requires a unique approach to care if professionals are to meet the wide variety of needs of the individual women and families. Cumberlege (1993) argues that,

'Pregnancy is a long and special journey for a woman and her family. It's a journey of dramatic physical, psychological and social change; of becoming a mother, of redefining family relationships; of taking the long-term responsibility of caring for, and cherishing a newborn child. Generations of women have travelled this same route; yet, each journey is unique'.

CHAPTER TWO

Psychological Theories Related to Practice

Psychological theories consist of five main approaches. Different theorists approach the study of mind and behaviour from different perspectives and consider particular aspects of an individual to be the most valuable in trying to understand the mind and behaviour of that individual.

There are five major approaches to the study of psychology. The most well-known is the psychodynamic or psychoanalytic theory of Sigmund Freud. Freud (Gross, 1992) suggests that the individual is made up of three elements of personality, the *Id*, the *Ego* and the *Superego*. The Id is the basic instinct or the pleasure principle. Its sole purpose is to satisfy basic needs and wants. The Ego is the reality principle which tries to meet the demands of the Id with what can actually be attained. The Superego is the conscience of the individual, which tries to temper the Id with what is acceptable within the normal social framework. These three elements are in conflict, each endeavouring to meet its own needs. Psychological normality exists when these elements are in some degree of harmony, and when in disharmony psychological ill-health ensues. Freud (Gross, 1992) argues that there are crucial stages in early psychosexual development during which the individual may encounter difficulties and unresolved issues which may affect subsequent psychological normality. It has to be remembered, however, that Freud's study was carried out on those individuals who had already presented with problems and not on 'normal' individuals

A second approach is the behaviourist one where only 'observable behaviour' is considered a means of assessing psychological status. The most widely known behaviourists are Watson and Skinner whose study was focused mainly on animals and argued that all behaviour is learned through some form of conditioning. Behaviour is reinforced either positively, to promote that behaviour, or negatively, to discourage that form of behaviour. Behaviourists would argue that all our normal social practices have been learned through conditioning, through the responses of significant others in the life of the developing individual, and the process continues throughout life. Behaviour is considered an important indicator of psychological wellbeing and is one which pervades all aspects of study.

The humanistic approach, put forward by Maslow and by Carl Rogers, is one which considers that self-development, knowledge and aesthetics are the most significant aspects of the individual. This approach, being client-centred, meets the current thinking in health care provision, which stresses the need for the client to maintain control over decisions which affect the self and to maintain her own self worth through collaboration with her carers.

The neurobiological approach considers that psychological ill-health is caused through biogenic malfunction or maladaption giving rise to psychological symptoms. Consequently, it is considered that physical treatments, e.g. chemotherapy can help relieve symptoms and regain normal patterns of behaviour.

The cognitive approach to the study of psychology is one in which the individual is considered to be an information processor. This is a relatively new perspective on the psyche of the individual and is allied to the development of the computer and of artificial intelligence. Cognitive psychology focuses on the internal mental processes (Gross, 1992), trying to understand the thought processes which have brought about a particular behaviour. This will include the beliefs and intentions of the individual. Cognitive psychology appears to be a progression of behavioural psychology in attempting to understand the mental processes which influences the decision-making abilities of the individual.

In clinical practice, no one approach is used in isolation. Practitioners may not always be conscious of the way in which they use their implicit knowledge of psychology to influence events. In daily life most of us make a very cursory but often fairly accurate assessment of another person with whom we are interacting. Health practitioners are no different, in that they too tend to 'label' and pigeonhole clients. They may not be conscious of the ways in which they employ 'layman's psychology' to assess individual clients, and this may influence the effectiveness of the communication which takes place. The professional may even employ subconscious techniques to encourage conformity in the client and to maintain control over care. The client may be encouraged to ask questions about her management, but the way in which a professional responds, in terms of both verbal and nonverbal response, can be directive and conforming. For example, a client may ask, 'Is an ultrasound safe?'. A professional may respond with, 'Oh, it's nothing to worry about – it's used all the time – you'll enjoy seeing your baby'. The professional has not answered the question, nor given any information about the examination with which the woman can make an informed choice. Instead the professional has offered empty reassurance, dismissed the question and closed the dialogue. In so doing, the professional has retained the expert knowledge, maintained the subservience of the questioner and possibly discouraged the questioner from asking for more information. The verbal response may also be accompanied by a lack of eye-contact which will further reduce the importance of the dialogue. It conveys to the client that neither she, nor the information seeking, is worthy of much attention. Usually the client will desist from pursing it, conform and have the examination. The 'Changing Childbirth' Report argues that 'women want improved information that allows them to make informed choices' (Cumberlege, 1993). An understanding of psychological theories can enable health practitioners to understand not only the client but also the impact that they have on the client's perception of care.

Personality

The term personality is one which has such broad general usage that it makes defining the term very difficult. In 1927 Allport identified 50 different definitions of the term. However, personality can be thought of as the central core of our psychological being. It is the difference between individuals; an aspect which cannot be ignored in any form of interaction. Personality is defined by Atkinson et al (1985) as 'the characteristic patterns of behaviour, thought and emotion that determine a person's adjustment to the environment'. The characteristic patterns of behaviour, thought and emotion are different within each of us but these are 'controlled' by what we have learned to be socially acceptable. There is a range of norms of behaviour and responses, which can be quite broad. However, when you look around a room *you* are the most normal person present! In other words, our norms are perceived from our own perspective. The term 'characteristic' implies that there is consistency in behaviour, so individuals usually respond within the framework of what is considered normal by the majority of the population. Personality affects how we interact with others and also how they will respond to us. It affects all areas of our interaction with others.

Personality is thought of mainly in the light of trait theories and type theories. These theories are used in everyday life to classify individuals whom we meet. We describe people in terms of traits if we describe them as warm, friendly, trustworthy and so on. We normally use this form of description of individuals whom we know relatively well. For those who are less well known to us we use type categories. These are broader classifications, such as extrovert, sociable. We make assessments of individuals as soon as we meet them. We do the same with clients and colleagues. Within seconds we have assessed whether or not we can relate easily to the new individual or whether some other approach is necessary to build the relationship and hence the confidence of the individual in us as a health professional. It must be remembered that our professional personality may be quite different from our private personality. We have a number of me's. These vary, depending on our social role at the time and there can be a conflict of these roles. All of this will affect our attitude, which is an essential part of our personality.

The study of personality can be approached in two ways – the ideographic approach and the nomothetic approach. The ideographic approach examines the behaviour, experiences and feelings of individuals. This approach studies the individual in depth. The nomothetic approach, on the other hand, looks at general laws which address the similarities and differences between people. Allport's approach was ideographic, looking at personality traits, whereas Eysenck's approach is a nomothetic one, looking at similarities and differences. Eysenck developed the theory of extrovert and introvert dimensions of personality

Eysenck's theory of personality looks at different types. 'Types' first appeared in Greek culture when Galen (129–199AD) claimed to have identified four 'humours' or body fluids – blood, bile, phlegm and black bile. These corresponded to personalities which were respectively sanguine (from the French sang meaning blood), a cheerful, optimistic type; choleric, an angry type; phlegmatic, a dull unresponsive type and melancholic, a sad gloomy type. These terms are still used today to describe individuals. Eysenck's classification to some extent correlated with these types. Using questionnaires to measure personality, Eysenck developed four dimensions of personality: introversion-extroversion and stable-neurotic. Within this framework, individuals can be classified into one of the four quadrants as a stable introvert or stable- extrovert, or neurotic introvert or neurotic extrovert.

Allport's (1961) notion was that personality is dynamic – always changing or being modified in the light of experiences. Allport defined personality as 'the dynamic organization within the individual of those psychological systems that determine his characteristics, behaviour and thought'. Personality is contained within the person, not in terms of social roles, but is built upon the notion of traits. These traits are responsible for how different people respond in the same situation. Traits are not present at birth and focus on conscious intentions. Traits can be divided into cardinal traits and central traits. Cardinal traits are all pervasive and are most influential, such as the trait of selflessness displayed by such persons as Florence Nightingale, Mother Teresa of Calcutta and others. Central traits identify characteristics, such as energy, reliability, capability. These traits are identified through observing consistent patterns of response.

Having an understanding of how our personality can influence both our approach to care and how the care we give is perceived by the client will enable us to be more open in recognizing our own shortcomings and limitations when dealing with different individuals. In recognizing that we cannot relate well to all individuals in our care it may be possible to address the issue with them so that we can care as well as possible within the limitation acknowledged. Alternatively we can suggest that another health professional might be able to meet the individual needs of the client to a higher degree and thus to give the client the optimum care possible whilst enabling the health professional to work within his or her own identified limitations. This should give the individual health professional a feeling of greater autonomy of practice and a higher level of job satisfaction.

Self, self-concept, self-image

The self is an integral part of the personality. Self-concept is defined by Stratton and Hayes (1993) as 'the sum total of ways in which the individual sees her or himself'. The self concept is considered to have two elements – the self-image and self-esteem. Self image has three aspects which influence it: self image as we are, self-image of how we would like to be and self-image as others perceive us. The self-image is in turn affected by our social roles of which we have many. For example we are daughters, sisters, wives, mothers, and we have professional roles which have a hierarchical structure and which influence how we react in any situation. We respond differently as wives from the way that we do as mothers and differently again in our professional roles. We use different language, different gestures and adopt different proximity to the person with whom we are communicating.

Self-esteem is defined by Stratton and Hayes (1993) as the personal evaluation which an individual makes of himself or herself; a sense of our own worth or capabilities. High self-esteem prompts a response of high regard, whereas low self-esteem prompts a response of low regard. How people feel about themselves affects their self-esteem and, as a consequence, affects how others respond to them. Try going into a shop to complain. For the first attempt you should be unkempt, using a limited vocabulary and using short or monosyllabic words. The second time, try complaining in a well-educated voice, using complex language structures and looking clean, fresh and professional. You will usually find that the responses to each approach are totally different. This premise also holds true when caring for clients. We tend to make an immediate assessment of their self-worth using similar criteria and may be surprised when the response we get is not that which is expected. This in turn affects our own feeling of self-worth.

Argyle (1969) suggests that there are four major factors which influence the self-concept. They are:

a)   reaction of others;
b)   comparison with others;
c)   social roles; and,
d)   identification.

Reaction to others is dependent on previous experience of others and the effect which our personality has on the other individual during the reciprocal interaction.

The self concept is important in care because our self concept affects how we care and the recipient's self concept affects how they respond to the care offered. Health professionals need to be aware of all the factors which influence their approaches to care. We try to treat all individuals sympathetically and professionally. However, we are all human and must recognize that we do not always meet the high standards of interaction for which we strive. Our self-esteem will be affected either positively or negatively by events which have preceded our interaction with the client. Some of these events may have occurred in the recent past, such as a reprimand from a superior which may have lowered our self-esteem or increased resentment. We may reflect this in our approach to a client, which consequently may not be as sensitive, or client focused, as it would normally be. Conversely, if we have just had an examination result in which we were successful, that too will affect our interaction. It may be that our self-esteem is so raised that we temporarily lose sight of the client's needs, or we respond to a very high standard which will be evident in response from the client. This reaction will further positively reinforce a high self-esteem.

The client will be similarly affected. If events which preceded her visit either positively or negatively affected her own self-esteem, then the health professional may continue that reinforcement positively or negatively and the interaction will either develop or fail.

The self concept, therefore, is a vital element of the interaction process. As health professionals, we need to be able to assess ourselves to identify the inhibitors and promoters of interaction which exist and to try to control the feelings which we have in order to offer the optimum care to the client. It is also necessary to identify in the client the difficulties she may be having in developing a rapport with her carer. A client who has a good rapport will have a very positive view of the quality of the care given, irrespective of the outcome of the care. If she feels that the health professionals had done their best in the most sensitive and empathic way possible, the client will be satisfied with the standard of care. If, however, there are inhibiting elements present during care, these will adversely affect the client's perception of the quality of the care she was given. Quality of care is a central issue and one which benefits both the client in terms of satisfaction with care and the health professional in terms of job satisfaction.

Attitude

Attitude is an aspect of our self which we display to others in all our interactions. Attitude may be defined as the way in which an individual responds to and influences events. Attitude relates to one's beliefs, values and norms and consequently will differ from individual to individual. The carer's attitude is a vital factor in the client's perception of the quality of care she receives, and may colour her whole experience of childbearing. One forgets that a client at all stages of childbearing needs reassurance that they are 'doing the right thing' for their baby. I was once cared for by a midwife who 'tutted' constantly and apart from being irritating, she gave me the impression that she was dissatisfied – both generally and with me in particular! Our attitude conveys approval, assurance, warmth, confidence and all that being 'with woman' is about. Caring for a client is a relatively intimate social interaction, the intimacy of which is usually established over a brief timeframe. This places the client in a vulnerable position and her vulnerability is increased if she is in labour. It is difficult to maintain self-esteem and assert oneself when in pain.

The poor attitude of a carer may be the result of a succession of unfortunate experiences on a given day. A colleague who witnesses the difficulties and traumas of a work period may well understand the carer's attitude. However, the client only has a restricted picture of events which have occurred; some events will be unknown to the client – all that the client experiences is the attitude of the carer towards *her*. The client will have had experiences which will have influenced her attitude prior to the encounter with the midwife, and which will influence her response. Heider (cited Spear, Penrod and Baker, 1988) argues that an imbalance in attitude often 'fosters a state of unpleasant tension'. The midwife needs to recognize that part of the role of carer is to foster a pleasant atmosphere in which relationships can grow.

The first meeting with a client is highly significant and it is important that the midwife establishes a good rapport through nonverbal communication such as appropriate eye contact, smile and possibly touch. This is not difficult in most circumstances, but when a client is in labour these reassuring techniques can be overlooked, particularly in a pressured situation. I often advise students that when talking to a client in labour it is important to ensure that they are making eye contact with the woman's *eyes* and not with her *vulva*! It is very disconcerting to have one's vulva spoken to and is not normal in any culture! However, health professionals do talk to various parts of a client's anatomy – I heard one client respond with a wave and say to the carer, 'I'm up here!'. The more aware we are as carers of the impact we have on the care given, then the more we are able to influence it positively. A client with a disastrous outcome will still say she has been given 'good care' if that care was sensitive, appropriate and responded to her emotional needs.

During labour a client is particular susceptible emotionally and the presence of pain increases that susceptibility. A client, therefore, needs to be shown warmth and consideration of *all* her needs in order that her individual needs are truly met.

Practitioners are encouraged to give individual care and most midwives would argue that they do give individual care, but that tends to be in the light of physical needs rather that psychological needs. As one learns more about the psychology of care, however, the better and more holistic care can be. Attitudes are a learned phenomenon and are learned through experience with a reference group or groups. In the case of health professionals, the reference group is normally one's peers and colleagues. Midwives themselves also have psychological needs in their very demanding work. All health professionals should adopt an approach of collaboration and cooperation in care, so that the needs of the carers are also addressed. Health professionals should avoid criticism of the care given by other health professionals, unless it is constructive and in the presence of the individual concerned.

Attitude, therefore, is a very important issue in care and one of which the midwife needs to be constantly aware. The client does not necessarily appreciate the difficulties that the midwife has encountered that day and it is not the client's concern. However, the midwife needs to be aware of the antecedents of all events pertaining to the client and also of how she, the midwife, may respond because of preceding events. The psychological wellbeing of the client is often largely dependent on the attitude of the carer.

Perception of control

Control is the ability to exert power and to influence the behaviour of others. Control can be exerted through several different avenues and can have a profound effect on the recipient by withdrawing or limiting their control over their own life event. Control, therefore, is a commodity which should be employed with caution in the field of health care and there should be serious consideration of the impact of that control.

Control can be exerted through the written word, the spoken word, through facial or bodily expressions, action or inaction. Control in childbearing is particularly important in relation to the woman's feeling of satisfaction with a traumatic and protracted life event. In most areas of our lives we control, to a large extent, what happens or does not happen to us. Our upbringing hinges on our gradually being given control over our lives as we mature towards adulthood. In a free society we are encouraged both to make and live with the important decisions in our lives and yet when it comes to one of the most important life events, childbearing, pregnant women appear to be considered by some health care professionals of being less capable of making decisions. It is often said by pregnant women that they feel that their bodies have become public property!

Even today, do *all* health care professionals on *every* occasion ask the woman's permission before touching her? Touching during childbearing is frequent and involves intimate touch. There are few occasions in life when a relative stranger strokes one's abdomen! This control and permission should remain with the woman. The reason for touching (albeit a professional examination of her condition) should always be given and permission gained prior to the examination and during the examination if necessary. It is often assumed that permission is unspoken simply by the woman arriving for her appointment! Of course. it is not only health professionals who touch pregnant women without permission. The public generally feel that pregnancy is a social event and will often ask a pregnant woman 'How are you keeping?' whilst at the same time stroking her abdomen. Stroking a woman's abdomen is not a usual form of greeting in any culture! Control of one's body and what happens to one's body is important and should not be taken over by some more knowledgeable professionals during childbearing.

Control can be mutual or distributed asymmetrically between carer and client. However, it is essential that control is negotiated so that each individual is clear about the process and procedure. It is necessary for the pregnant woman so that her psychological needs are met and for the professional so that their professional integrity and credibility is maintained. It must be remembered that negotiation is a two-way discussion – a dialogue, involving exchange of information and a consensus being reached which satisfies all parties. Negotiation is not only the verbal exchange but also the nonverbal communication and behaviour. Wiemann (1985) stresses the importance of nonverbal communication and the making of control moves or bids which may be accepted or challenged. A woman should be encouraged to maintain control by questioning processes and procedures and by the health professional adopting a relaxed approach which is non-threatening to the woman. It is also important that the professional does not undermine a woman's control by addressing her too informally before that stage in the relationship is reached. The balance of control may be influenced by a number of factors including the social status of the woman, her dress, her vocabulary, her accent, or her use of 'medical' phrases. Equally a professional may remove control from a client by means of the same factors!

Negotiation and the maintenance of control is relatively easy in situations where there is a low rate of intimacy, but becomes increasingly difficult if an intimate examination is being conducted.

Many women find it difficult to assert themselves in any circumstances but consider how much more difficult is it for a woman who is lying down and not wearing her knickers. Negotiation should, therefore, take place before a woman prepares herself to be examined and whilst she is in an upright position, which is normal for most social exchanges.

A woman needs to feel in control during the childbearing process in order to ensure that not only her physical but also her psychological needs are met. The health professional can help a woman maintain control by assisting her, answering her in a friendly and sensitive way and bearing in mind how threatened and unsure the pregnant woman may feel. It is important that the empathic midwife encourages and supports the woman without undermining the woman's confidence in herself. Control in childbearing is a shared concept with the woman maintaining control over her body and what happens to it and the professional maintaining control over the professional issues of care as identified in Rules 40, 41 and 42 of the Midwives Rules (1993) emcompassing the legal duty of care and the maintenance of a safe environment.

CHAPTER THREE

Psychological Changes during Childbearing

There are considerable psychological adjustments which a pregnant woman has to make during her pregnancy. The changes which are occurring in her own body may cause stress and even distress. A woman's body image is often an important factor in her self-esteem. It is known that overweight women often have a mental body image of the slim women they once were. As pregnancy progresses, a woman may find the change of body shape a comforting image, but for others it will be more distressing as the pregnancy progresses, particularly if the pregnancy is unwanted, unexpected or unwelcome. Her partner, in his response to the pregnancy, may also positively or negatively affect her response and her psychological adjustment.

The main anxiety which a woman experiences during pregnancy is whether or not she is carrying a normal fetus. Several tests are carried out by professionals in order to assess normality of the fetus. In reality, they are attempting to exclude abnormality and, as a result, any antenatal test can increase anxiety during pregnancy. Professionals may not be aware of the anxiety levels of their clients nor of how an assessment affects the client. The majority of assessments are carried out with only cursory explanations and the safety of such assessments tends to be assumed, which may or may not be justified.

There are adjustments to be made within the family structure as women move from their daughter/partner role to their role of potential mother. Their antecedent sexual activity is now a matter of public knowledge, where it was formerly private. This change causes increased stress due to the perceived expectations of the role both by the individual woman and also by the wider family. These expectations may well differ between individuals and without effective communication within the family tensions may increase. Social pressures encourage conformity of behaviour which is not necessarily what a woman and her partner may wish. It is often difficult for a couple to carry out their wishes and desires because of the social pressures imposed on them. This is made more difficult within some cultures because the 'rules' are implicit and not an issue for discussion.

Anxiety may also be increased due to the type of work carried out by the woman. She may require a modification of her role at work in order to accommodate the pregnancy. There is also the financial stress which occurs during a pregnancy. There are additional costs and anxiety about coping financially after the birth.

It should be remembered that professionals also influence a woman's attitude to her pregnancy. Chance remarks can cause great offence, such as a woman expecting her fourth child who was asked 'Do you *really* want this baby?' The assumption being that once the prescribed 'pigeon pair' has been achieved, then anything else is excessive or the result of failed contraception!

Guilt may also play a part in pregnancy, either because the pregnancy was unplanned or ill-timed, or because of the increased demands which will be made on both partners. Lifestyle is also given close consideration and women particularly feel guilty if they continue to smoke during pregnancy. These women need to be given positive feedback about what they are, or have achieved, and not criticized for their lack of achievement.

Health professionals should take care with both what they say to a pregnant woman and also how they say it, and remember that their role is to offer care and advice to the pregnant woman and her family and to ensure that physical and psychological wellbeing is promoted and maintained.

Psychological preparation for parenthood

Parenthood is an event which has a relatively sudden onset and the condition tends to be lifelong! Sylvia Plath wrote in her poem entitled *Metaphors,* 'I've boarded the train there's no getting off'. Preparation for parenthood begins in our own childhood with the example of our parents. As children we engage in role play and symbolic interaction and from that learn how to cope with fictitious situations, often mimicking our parents. However, parenting is not an undemanding state and for some individuals it can be extremely difficult. It is not an innate response and for most individuals parenting is learned through trial and error. Consequently it can be emotionally traumatic when caring for a new family member is found to be more difficult than anticipated.

Parenthood – and motherhood in particular – is a life crisis for which one is never really prepared. A new mother has to cope with tiredness, physical changes, lactation, soreness and – the aspect which can be most distressing – leaking from so many orifices! This causes a problem with maintaining the standard of hygiene that the woman is used to. A number of women also find the smell of milk unpleasant and as a new mother it is difficult to escape it.

Mothers will each respond differently to their new role. The individual's ability to cope will affect her ability to interact with her infant. However, early mother–infant interaction increases the mother's confidence in her ability to care effectively for her infant. Gottman (1956) argued that, in order to perform a new role effectively, the newcomer puts on a mask. The new mother tries to give the impression of possessing the necessary qualities for parenting and this in itself is stressful. This transition is part of the preparation for the new role and in a sense parents never complete the transition, since parenting is both dynamic and organic and is constantly changing and throwing up new problems. The new mother not only has to cope with her baby, but also with her role adjustment from partner/wife to mother and to the demands which the wider family may make of her in terms of cultural and/or social issues, such as a religious ritual, which need to be addressed.

The lack of quality sleep combined with the unfamiliar demands increases stress levels and may make the mother tearful and adversely affect her ability to cope. Her sense of her own inadequacy may also be increased by the competent professional, who will often bath or change the infant in a fraction of the time which it takes a new mother to carry out the tasks. The professional is also often very good at 'settling' the baby when it is fretful. It is important to remember whose baby it is and that the mother's confidence is built through supporting her in care. It can be helpful when one parent is unsure of an aspect of care if the partner carries it out and together they work out *their* best way of coping. Parents often try to be 'perfect', to achieve the ideal, but it should be stressed that so long as the infant is clean, warm and fed and the mother is the same that they are coping well. It is OK to be 'good enough'.

It is also not uncommon for new mothers not to like their infants. This may sound strange, but few mothers are confident enough to admit it. They do not necessarily get the baby they ordered; they get the one that was delivered which may not quite meet their expectations. It may look like an unfavourite relative or it may be particularly difficult to feed or settle. A newborn infant does not reciprocate very much for all the attention it is given and some parents find parenting *very boring!* Many individuals would consider that it is not culturally acceptable to admit to feeling unhappy as a new mother. In helping a new parent in their psychological adjustment, the professional carer needs to lower their expectations and minimize the advice that they offer whilst encouraging the new parent to feel free to ask as many questions as they want. It should be remembered that the first days and weeks in any new job are very stressful and an individual may consider handing in their notice. This option is not available to new parents and so they need extra support and consideration to cope with the massive adjustments which they are making, at a time when they person creating the readjustment is unrelenting in their demands. The couple also need time to adjust to their relationship and to find time to be together and resume normal marital relations before the child starts at University!

Stress related to childbearing

Stress is a subject which has become an issue of great concern in recent years both in society as a whole, but also in the health professions. Stress is now known to be a contributory factor in a number of illnesses and can, if not dealt with, adversely affect the outcome of an illness or, indeed, lead to an illness. Stress is experienced by all members of society. The *Oxford English Dictionary* defines stress as 'the overpowering pressure of some adverse force or influence'. This definition suggests a loss of control or of an issue being beyond the control of the individual. Childbearing may sometimes be seen as a loss of personal control and a 'taking over' of one's body for the purpose of producing a child. Certainly, in early pregnancy there is a sense of detachment from the 'baby', of the unreality of the situation in which a woman finds herself. This may be attributed to the 'time-lag' between the loving act of sexual intercourse and the confirmation of the pregnancy.

There are two types of stress – positive and negative stress – which can affect how the individual reacts. A positive stress is one which motivates, drives and gives satisfaction, whereas a negative stress is one which demands, taxes and drains the individual. Stress is different in different circumstances.

There is also intrinsic stress and extrinsic stress. Intrinsic stress relates to an individual's personal goals, their striving for perfection in areas of private and professional life. It is important to many individuals to achieve and maintain a high standard in all or most areas of their life, and to some extent society reinforces this idea by encouraging the social norms which help to maintain a stable society. Difficulties arise when the norms and values are challenged and changes are made. A good example of this is single parenthood, which was frowned upon socially half a century ago, and by some individuals still is, but the majority of society accepts single parenthood and also accepts that people have a right to choose the way they live their lives. The feeling of self-worth comes from not only how we feel about ourselves but also from how our partners feel about us.

Extrinsic stress is brought about by external factors, such as pain, bereavement, loneliness and childbearing.

Stress during childbearing can be attributed to three aspects as highlighted by Burnard (1991):

a)   stress within the individual;
b)   stress caused by others (the health professionals, family);
c)   stress caused by the pressure of society to conform.

Stress from within the individual can be related to the anxiety regarding her ability to cope with the demands of pregnancy and labour, her ability to produce a normal healthy infant and her ability to maintain her own self-esteem throughout a traumatic and rapidly changing time in her life. The change in the woman's social role from an independent person to one who is dependent on others, i.e. the health professional, in a field where the language may be alien and to some degree threatening in the sense that not everything uttered is fully understood without further inquiry, may exacerbate the woman's stress and feeling of being in control of events. The 'Changing Childbirth' Report (1993) is enabling women to exert their right to choose. The report states,

> 'The woman must be the focus of maternity care. She should be able to feel that she is in control of what is happening to her and able to make decisions about her care, based on her needs, having discussed matters fully with the professionals involved'.

Stress can affect an individual in many areas. There can be physical signs of stress, such as excessive tiredness; cognitive signs of stress, such as lack of concentration, memory difficulties; and emotional signs such as tearfulness, over-anxiety and all of these will have some impact on the outward behaviour of the individual. Negative stress may result in lower self-esteem. Self-esteem relates to the way in which we regard ourselves and self-esteem may differ in varying situations. When an individual feels vulnerable, their self-esteem is threatened and consequently they may react in an over-assertive way, by demanding and arguing or, more usually they will adopt a submissive role, where they will not challenge what is happening to them, and so are perceived by the carer as being 'cooperative clients'. This 'cooperation' may simply be a coping mechanism for the present, which will ultimately contribute to the negative stressors which will undermine the woman's self confidence.

Coping mechanisms vary with individuals, but physical ways of coping will often dissipate stress. Taking an active interest in a hobby, or exercising, will relieve tension. Self-nurture is an area about which some women feel guilty, but to take time for yourself in an important part of maintaining a healthy self. Allowing enough time for rest is not always achievable. Equally a well-balanced diet is difficult to maintain for some individuals, but is especially important in childbearing. Giving oneself 'treats' can be very positive for de-stressing the individual.

A method which most people find valuable is emotional expression. By talking and sharing concerns and anxieties, it can often serve to relieve the anxiety in some measure. Women will cry more readily than men and in that way release tension-relieving chemicals in to the circulation. Some individuals may find an artistic outlet more valuable, such as poetry, art or music.

Confronting the problem of stress is a useful technique and enables the individual to take control of the issue. In childbearing, control of care is slowly being transferred to the woman through the use of informed choice. Women are being encouraged to be assertive, to know their rights and know how to use the present system of care to benefit themselves most. It is important that the individual also is aware of the expectations and limitations of others. In order to keep stress levels to a minimum it is important to maintain a balance in all aspects of life. This can be achieved during the childbearing process through discussion and negotiation, so that the needs of the woman, her family and the demands of the health care professions are met to a large degree.

CHAPTER FOUR

The Psychology of Pain

The word pain comes from the Latin word *poena* meaning punishment in the form of physical or mental suffering. Pain is also a warning signal that something is amiss, that there is damage, and damage or injury needs to be dealt with. Labour causes considerable pain but this pain is productive rather than destructive. However, knowing this does not necessarily make it any easier to bear! Spear, Penrod and Baker (1988) argue that pain is a complex sensory experience which can produce both sensory and emotional response. Pain perception is extremely variable in individuals and there are cases of women giving birth with relatively little pain. It is also true that some women appear to experience quite severe pain from the onset of labour. This variation in the way in which different individuals perceive pain is usually related to past experience, memory, their ability to cope with pain and their culture. Postle (1988) suggests that if experience of life is pain free, then one copes constructively. If life has been good enough one perseveres stubbornly, influenced by many factors such as anxiety, uncertainty, fatigue, depression and even the time of day. Pain often appears worse at night when limited help is available, whereas in daylight when there is an ability to do something about the pain if often does not seem so bad. Attitudes to pain also vary as does the extent to which one is prepared for pain. A pregnant woman was heard to say that she was not ready mentally for labour today. Preparation is an important part of the coping mechanism for pain. An individual who is being assertive keeps the pain in control and tends to dominate the pain. However, if an individual is already tired from emotional pressure, then they tend to become submissive to that pain and the pain dominates.

The attitude of the professional is also an important factor in a client's pain perception. The professional may regard pain as a symptom which requires treatment or a side effect which requires monitoring, as a normal physiological function. Health professionals feel that their role is to alleviate pain, but this is in order to relieve the client, or to relieve the stress it causes a carer to see a client in pain?

Prince and Adams (1987) recognized that 'subjective experience of pain has no direct relationship to the extent of physical trauma'. It has to be acknowledged that, if a client is describing moderate or severe pain, then they are indeed experiencing that pain and they should not be assessed in the light of how others have coped in a similar situation. This is because although the physical situation may be similar the psychological situation may be very different, as each woman has a different emotional framework, within which the pain is experienced. Baron and Byrne (1991) suggest that when a person has confidence in his or her ability, the body releases natural painkillers which enhance performance and reduce stress. It is important, therefore, that a woman is encouraged and supported during labour, in order to enable her to cope positively with the pain she experiences. It is also important that the environment should be warm, comfortable, relaxing and allow the woman the freedom to sit, stand, walk and dress as she wishes. A woman would normally have this freedom of choice in her own home, but convention dictates that, when in a strange environment (as, for example, in a maternity unit), one adopts a conformity of behaviour which is socially acceptable, but which is not necessarily the behaviour which enables a woman to cope with pain.

The role of the professional health carer is to prepare by giving well-researched information on pain and its relief; by adopting a non-judgemental approach to pain when caring; to build confidence, explain and reassure as the labour progresses. A health professional who is empathic, sensitive, open, honest and well informed is one who offers the best quality of care to a client. It is often not the actual care given, but the way in which the care is delivered, that influences the perception of the quality of care. Pain is part of labour and the ability to cope with pain is dependent upon the relationships between carer and client. An understanding of the ways in which a client describes her pain and of the background and culture of the client, will enable the professional to help the client with the psychological demands of pain and of the labour process.

The psychological impact of birth

The psychological changes which a woman undergoes following the birth process are not normally given much consideration. However, if a person were to have an operation and then were asked to start a new job the following day most people would find this unreasonable. Motherhood is different, since this is exactly what is asked of a woman.

Many individuals consider childbirth as a normal physiological event, which, of course, it is. But it is not a hourly, daily, weekly or monthly event like most other physiological processes and therefore demands more of the individual. For some women the event is so traumatizing that they never want to repeat it! Childbearing is not easy, physically or psychologically. A woman needs nurturing, understanding and supporting to enable her to cope with the excessive demands of early motherhood. It has to be remembered that a woman is also suffering sleep deprivation following birth. This deprivation is not simply that which occurred during labour, but has often built up over the many preceding months. This may be due to a number of factors, such as the physical discomfort of the expanding abdomen, breast tenderness, increased bladder activity, heartburn and leg cramps. It is also usual that when a mother settles down to rest, it appears to be a signal for her fetus to start practising footballing techniques or to try bracing itself against the bed. Sleep deprivation, therefore, is a very real consideration after birth. It impairs a woman's ability to think logically, argue reasonably or plan coherently and is worse in some women than in others. Yet a woman is usually expected to get up the morning after delivery and care competently for her infant!

The impact of birth is also influenced by the type of labour and the length of that labour as well as the care a woman has been given. In a labour where a woman perceives that she was in control and where there has been a satisfactory outcome for the mother and family, the woman will normally feel better able to cope with the demands following labour.

It should be remembered that a woman may not have got the baby she wanted. It may be the wrong sex, the wrong hair colouring, the wrong temperament and the mother will be affected by the way in which her baby behaves. Mothers often have a mental image of the ideal infant and newborns rarely meet that ideal. Newborns are, after all, individuals who may be quiet or noisy, placid or demanding, have large or small appetites and be cooperative or uncooperative. A mother is expected to cope with all of this. Along with the infant, the mother is also coping with a variety of physical discomforts. She may have perineal pain or discomfort, breast pain or discomfort, and/or abdominal pain or discomfort. The woman also has personal expectations of her own ability to cope with motherhood and she is now in the limelight, with partner, mother, mother-in-law and other family members watching her caring for her infant. Most individuals do not perform well when being watched critically by others!

It should also be remembered that the new infant may not be the woman's only responsibility, particularly if it is a multiple birth. The woman may have other children at home needing care, and even pets need special attention following the arrival of a new family member. Western society tends to expect a woman to return to normal household chores within days of delivery and, surprisingly, a lot of women achieve this. This is only a social norm because we allow it to be. Women should decide what is right for them, and not allow themselves to be pressured by others into behaving in a socially prescribed way. If a woman is encouraged to gain as much physical and psychological rest as she needs, she will recover more quickly from any trauma experienced during the birth process. This requires understanding and support from the family and from professionals.

A woman often needs to talk through the birth process with someone who will listen sensitively. This is part of the healing process and enables the woman to come to terms with the labour and delivery. This role can be filled by a professional, or by a member of the family who has both the time and the listening skills.

The birth process has a significant psychological impact on the woman, but with an empathic approach to care by both health professionals and the wider family any woman can face the transition to motherhood without trepidation. Hopefully, she will also get more enjoyment and personal satisfaction from the experience of early mothering.

CHAPTER FIVE

Neonatal Perceptions and Abilities

The ability of the newborn to interact with its environment is important for its survival. The human baby is one of the most helpless of all infants in the animal kingdom. Darwin, in 1872, was one of the first to document the infant's smile as a 'strong social signal'. The smile is often thought of as the first sign of communication which takes three to six weeks to develop (Wolff, 1963). However, there are many other ways in which a newborn infant affects its environment. At delivery, the infant usually makes its presence felt by crying – to the parents delight and that of the health professionals who assist the delivery. It signals that the infant is alive and hopefully normal. The sociability of the infant is mainly targeted at satisfying its basic need for food, warmth and love. Crying is highly likely to be followed by maternal interaction. Moss (1967) and Wolff (1969) identified three distinct types of cry, signalling hunger, pain and anger, which the mother can differentiate between by the time the infant is three months of age. Schaffer (1977) suggests that infants acquire an understanding of their effect on their environment. The experience of health practitioners and parents supports this view.

Crying is one of several means of interaction. The infant can also make eye contact, gesture, listen and babble and imitate. The infant is very alert after delivery and spends time scanning his or her new environment, and, if the mother opts to breastfeed at this time her infant will engage in eye contact. Breastfeeding lends itself to early and prolonged mother-infant interaction owing to the fact that the distance from eye to breast, approximately 20cm (8"), matches the focusing ability of the newborn (Schaffer, 1977).

Fantz in 1961 highlighted the infant's ability to make sustained eye contact and also the infant's preference for looking at the human face. He suggests that this preference is innate. However, Hershenson (1967) argues that this is a 'learned preference'. The nature/nurture debate is a long and so far unresolved controversy.

The infant's listening skills can be observed in the early days of life. There is evidence that the fetus can hear from 24 weeks of pregnancy. Pregnant women will remark on how the fetus will 'jump' when a loud noise is suddenly experienced. In the early days of life if the mother holds her newborn's face close to her and talks to it, it will respond with babbles. The adult tends to match the conversation with the infants noises. This is part of the 'meshing behaviour' which has been written about by Stern (1977), and which also involves synchronized head movements and imitation of facial expressions. How often have we watched babies copying us when we poke our tongues out! We, of course, give positive reinforcement by praising them or laughing with them.

Bowlby (1984) and Winnicott (1964) argue that the infant cannot be studied in isolation and needs to be studied with its mother or primary caregiver. It is now acknowledged that the father and close family also play a large part in the normal development of an infant.

Babbling can heard from four weeks of age (Wolff, 1963) and by six weeks of age the babbling can last 10–15 minutes. It is also recognized that in the first six months of life an infant's babbling contains all the sounds of all the languages known to man and that in the second six months of life these sounds are restricted to those heard by the infant. It is, therefore, important for the carers to talk constructively to the child in order to promote normal development.

Theories of bonding and interaction

Bonding is a term which is used to describe the attachment felt by one person to another. Attachment is defined by Stratton and Hayes as,

> 'a close, emotionally meaningful relationship between two people in which each seeks closeness with the other and feels more secure in their presence'.

This describes the normal feelings which an individual feels for someone they love and wish to protect. Bowlby (1984) describes this feeling as being 'innately monotropic', that is an inborn feeling of attachment to one person usually the mother or 'primary caregiver' and that this tie is different with other people. However, Rutter (1991) argues that 'most children develop bonds with several people... and that the bonds are basically similar'. This emotional tie is normally reciprocal, that is felt by both individuals – they feel for each other.

Ainsworth et al (1978) in her study of the 'strange situation' highlights the feeling of loss which a child feels when its mother leaves its presence. It can be seen that is a two way effect. Therefore, when looking at attachment behaviour, the child cannot be studied in isolation from its mother, the two need to be studied together.

It is worth considering whether at the time of delivery the mother experiences this 'swoop of maternal love'. Most women expect this feeling but not all experience it. Most first-time mothers need time for the love for their infant to grow and develop. Initially the mother is grateful that the labour is over, she has coped with it and hopefully has a normal child. However, it may take several days or weeks for the love to develop and most mothers are reluctant to admit this lack of love for fear of being labelled by health professionals as inadequate or a potential risk to her infant. A self-confident mother once disclosed after several years that when her first child was born she did not feel love for it. After five weeks she confided in her own mother (who had had 12 children and had an excellent relationship with all her children) that she did not love her baby. Her mother smiled and replied, 'My dear, I didn't love any of you at first, but give it time'. The young mother was relieved and started to relax and think of her feelings as normal and then the love for her baby grew. It is often not until the infant makes a more conscious response to its mother, such as a smile at three to six weeks that the mother feels the warmth of love towards her infant.

Bonding thwarted

Health professionals often act as role models for new parents particularly first-time parents. It is obvious therefore that the way in which we behave towards the newborn is very important. Inexperienced health professionals may carry out a procedure on the infant without ever talking or explaining to the baby what is happening. This approach makes the assumption that the infant lacks any sensitivity or understanding and if parents emulate this approach the infant may suffer. Kochavenich-Wallace et al (1988) suggest that 'the treatment of parents and infants by hospital staff may affect parental feelings and attitudes'.

DeCasper and Fifer (1980) demonstrated that infants can not only distinguish their own mother's voice but also show a preference for hearing it. It is often difficult or embarrassing for a new mother to try to hold a 'conversation' with her baby but it is important to encourage her to do so by example. After all, the mother may well have been talking to her fetus during pregnancy and the infant is used to hearing her. Of course, a woman's mothering behaviour will often relate to her experience of being mothered or in the social setting of mothering – her sisters or other relatives demonstrating mothering skills. This experience is often more lasting that any skill taught by health professionals because it is more constant.

Separation

Separation of the newborn infant from the family, for example, when the newborn requires care in an Neonatal Unit, affects not only the infant, who lacks the closeness of its mother and the early nurturing which is the normal pattern of care, but it also affects the mother quite dramatically as well as the father and wider family.

The mother may experience a variety of feelings including inadequacy, believing she has failed in her primary role of mothering, confusion over the possible outcome of the separation, and she may also be emotionally labile. A mother needs to be near her infant following birth in order to reinforce the reality of having become a mother by exploring her infant to assess normality and family likenesses and to spend time developing this new relationship. Separation deprives a mother of this early interaction.

Animal studies (carried out by Lorenz (1935)) showed that there is a critical period for the formation of emotional attachments. However, this does not seem to be the case in humans. Rutter (1981) argues that adverse early life experiences do not necessarily have serious effects on the child. It seems that humans have a particular resilience to such events. However, privation of attachment may adversely affect the child's development, particularly the development of intelligence, language and social skills (Gross, 1992), but there is evidence of rapid recovery if the right environment is subsequently provided for the child. Older infants demonstrate clear effects of separation as shown in the study carried out by Ainsworth (1971), who examined the 'strange situation' and showed that infants had formed attachments to their primary care giver and showed grief at separation from them.

Mothers may also suffer a form of grief during separation from their infant. The emotional trauma of not being able to hold and care for one's newborn infant should not be underestimated and health professionals can support mothers by encouraging participation in care and enabling mothers to develop some interaction with even the most sick infants. There may even be the fear for the death of the infant in the mother's mind, which may inhibit her from allowing the relationship to develop. This is a form of self-protection to guard against some of the acute pain which the mother will experience if the infant does not survive or if it survives but is handicapped.

The father also has psychological needs during a stressful period. He has encountered dramatic changes in his life and may feel utterly helpless in a situation which is beyond his perceived control. Health professionals need to be empathic towards him, and explain events surrounding the separation of his infant in a language which is familiar to him. The majority of individuals are unfamiliar with hospital procedures, jargon, etiquette and norms and therefore it can be very difficult for a stranger to make informed choices about care when they have only a limited idea of the options. The use of familiar words without being patronizing is helpful, explaining terms which may not be familiar. This approach to care will help to build confidence in the affected relatives and also give them a measure of control.

The wider family

The grandparents and brothers and sisters of the infant are likewise distanced from the baby by enforced separation. Although the family normally fully understands the reason for the separation – because the infant needs closer observation or treatment – nevertheless the feeling of loss is still dramatic. Think of a young child excited by the addition to the family who then has restricted access to the baby. Restricted access is not being able to care for and explore the newborn as the sibling or grandparent normally would. They all want to hold and talk to the infant to reinforce the reality of the situation, for which they have waited for so long, has arrived. The disappointment and increased anxiety is almost inevitable and for some there will also be guilt. They may consider an event or action which they did may have contributed in some way to the baby not being 'perfect'. It is important, therefore that health professionals have an understanding of the mixed emotions which the wider family feels and be able to support and encourage them in their aspect of caring for the new family member.

Sibling rivalry

Sibling rivalry is a normal response by a child or children to the threat imposed on the stability of their family relationships by the newcomer. Sibling rivalry persists throughout life. Children continually vie for the attention of one or other of their parents. This rivalry shows itself in a variety of ways. The child may become more clinging or more detached. He or she may become more independent of the parent, but it is more common for them to revert to more childish behaviour, such as imitating a crying baby, or wanting to be bottle fed. A child who is toilet trained may start to wet or soil because, although this causes displeasure and anxiety on the part of the parent, it also enables the child to gain considerable attention from the parent. Time has to be spent consoling, cleaning and generally nursing the child. Other measures may be taken by the child to attract and retain the attention of the parent. This is particularly effective if the child is antisocial in its behaviour by being destructive of toys and other objects or, even more effectively, by throwing a tantrum! There are an infinite number of ways of irritating a parent if a child puts his or her mind to it! This is especially obvious when the parent is, or is about to be, involved in some aspect of baby care. It should be remembered that the child may not necessarily be jealous of the new baby but it may well be jealous of the time and attention given to the baby.

It is important that parents and professionals remember to include the other child or children in the care of the infant. It makes the young child or children feel important and useful. It also assures the child that there is a clear place for him or her in the new situation. Fathers can also experience a form of jealousy which is why it is important to include all family members in the care of the new infant. The professional should encourage positive interaction and it is valuable to ask other family members about the progress of the newborn. Even a two-year old can comment on the baby's progress.

A new member of the family affects the relationships of all the family members and older siblings usually take on new roles and behaviours. These behaviours can be reinforced through positive feedback to the child or the behaviour can be modified through negative feedback. An older child will usually enjoy the responsibility of helping to care for the newborn, but time needs to be set aside for the older child when the infant is asleep. Health professionals can help the older child with the adaptation, by including the child in the discussion of care, but it is important to listen to the child's response and help to diffuse some of the sibling rivalry which is an inevitable part of life.

Psychological impact of death

Death is an inevitable outcome of life, but when two stressful life events happen in close proximity to one another the effect is compounded. Birth normally has the effect of making the individuals concerned with the event feel elated. They feel great happiness and the sense of a new beginning and a new purpose in life. Death has completely the opposite effect. It reminds an individual of his own mortality and how brief and tenuous life really is. When birth and death occur around the same time there is usually an overwhelming feeling of loss and sadness. The purpose of life is questioned and there is often questioning of an individual's religious belief.

The Health Education Council statistics show that 6,000 babies die each year in the United Kingdom around the time of birth. Death around the time of birth cannot be considered uncommon. Consider the large number of individuals affected by these deaths each year and one realizes how important it is for health professional to have an understanding of the grieving process in order to offer some support to individuals or families who need it.

Grief is defined by Parkes and Weiss (1983) as, 'a normal reaction to overwhelming loss, albeit a reaction in which normal functioning no longer holds'. Individuals find it extremely difficult to function normally following a death. Berryman (1989) argues that death 'has been shown to have a particularly powerful effect on health'. She goes on to suggest that the levels of morbidity and mortality are raised in surviving relatives. It is not really surprising when one considers how attention and concentration are affected by such a life crisis.

The grieving process is not a rigid progression of events. Each individual will respond differently over time and gradually learn to live with their loss. Kubler-Ross (1970) identifies five stages of grief; denial, anger, bargaining, depression and acceptance. Engel (1962) discusses three phases of grief: disbelief, developing awareness and resolution. What is evident is that all theorists agree that grief has to be 'worked through'. Although Hinton (1975) suggests that the more severe mental pain will ease within a few weeks, Marris (1958) suggests that the *majority* of individuals are still distressed one year later.

Parkes and Weiss (1983) suggest that there are two issues which will complicate the grief process. The first is the mode of death – if it is sudden or unexpected the shock experienced is likely to be greater and more lengthy. The second is that society assumes there is a moral duty to grieve. The grief process can become abnormal if, as Bowlby suggests, the grief is unresolved, or absent.

Individuals need privacy to grieve. That does not mean isolation. It is important that they have support of loved ones and most importantly have a listening ear – someone who is prepared actively to listen to the feelings of the bereaved person over and over again. It is this repetition that helps an individual to come to terms with the loss and to understand why they feel as they do and that the feelings they are experiencing are *normal*. It is quite a worry for some bereaved individuals that they feel detached from the world around them and that they are 'going mad', particularly if they have said or done something which others might consider bizarre. One family took photographs of the funeral; it was their way of coming to terms with the loss.

Close relatives and friends often find it very difficult to know how to react to death and particularly what to say to the parents of a child who has died. It is often easier for friends to say nothing, but this can be very hurtful to the parents who may see it as a failure to acknowledge their baby. Simply saying, 'I'm sorry' is enough for the parents to accept that the friend is also feeling for them. Practically, it is useful for friends and relatives to be close by to carry out the ordinary everyday tasks for the bereaved couple. Make sure that they have something to eat or that there is milk for tea. Simple things, but sometimes the parent is so distressed for several weeks that they cannot cope with even the most ordinary events of life. This form of caring can be very demanding on the relative or friend who is also grieving, not necessarily for the lost baby but for the sadness that the loss has brought on their loved one.

It is important to remember that it is not just death which brings about a bereavement situation. Loss and grief is also experienced in situations of miscarriage, abortion and infertility, as well as the birth of a handicapped child. Parents or mothers who put their child forward for adoption may also feel grief and loss. This is particularly so if family pressure has been put on the mother to consider adoption, even though she may feel that it is in the best interests of the child. Finally, an event which causes tremendous conflict of emotions is in the case of a multiple birth where not all the infants survive. The parents may feel elation at the birth but desolation at the loss which may affect how they interact with the surviving child or children.

Health professionals need to help individuals through the grief process. They can do this by helping to create memories of the baby through talking and showing genuine concern. Always remember that parents are particularly sensitive to inappropriate remarks and that each death is unique. Parkes (1972) suggests that, 'getting over it doesn't mean forgetting or replacing – it is learning to live with the loss – it is always there'.

CHAPTER SIX

Psychological Needs of the Childbearing Woman

Both class and culture have individual social norms to which a member is expected to conform if they wish to remain an accepted part of that class or culture.

Class is a social division which has increasingly become eroded in recent years, in that the middle class culture has been subdivided into an upper and lower middle class. There are far more women in paid employment and, in fact, carrying out two jobs – one in paid employment and the other in unpaid employment in the home. Caring for the house and family is still primarily the role of the woman, despite the evolution of the 'modern man'. The woman still feels responsible for almost all household tasks and child care. This causes considerable emotional pressure, particularly if the woman also holds a demanding job. The additional pressure of pregnancy and childbearing exacerbates the stress of matching all the demands made of her. A woman feels guilty just for being a woman! The support of family and friends is an essential element of balancing all the demands. Increasingly nowadays, however, families do not stay in close knit communities, but live some distance apart making the family support networks difficult to maintain. This is made worse by the modern view of childbearing as being a 'normal physiological process', meaning that a woman can readily have her baby and continue all aspects of life as before. The reality is that the woman feels isolated and is often overawed by the responsibility of caring for a newborn baby, whether supported by a partner of not. Health professionals reinforce this view and generally give the woman little time to recover, both physically and psychologically, from what is a normal, physiological process but is also a major life event. Health professionals need to increase their awareness of the impact of childbearing and encourage and support the woman during the early parenting days.

Social pressure exists to encourage individuals to conform. This is especially strong from family members and from peers. Although, health professionals offer advice on baby care this may be superseded by advice from family and friends. It is not that the advice from family and friends is incorrect but it is not normally research-based. Feeding regimes and techniques are areas of particular concern and where women feel that they have received conflicting advice. Health professionals should encourage the woman to discuss the family's views on child care so that the issues and cultural variances can be evaluated by both the parents and the professionals, in order that the most practical decisions can be made for that family. Cultural influences and rites are often quite rigid around childbirth and it is important to recognize the value of the differing ways in which various cultures support and nurture the newly delivered mother. In some Indian cultures it is forbidden for the new mother to enter the kitchen because she is 'unclean'. The woman is cared for by the wider family for several weeks before she resumes her household tasks. This time enables the new mother to have the rest she needs and to spend time getting to know her new child. Many British born women would value the opportunity of such care, but Western culture tends to encourage the woman to 'get back to normal' as quickly as possible. As a result, by six weeks postpartum the new mother has reached the 'zombie' stage! Cultural and class differences should be encompassed into the plan of care for the family to enable as smooth a transition into parenthood as is possible whilst respecting the values and norms of that family.

Role of the midwife

The midwife has a unique role to play in the care and management of a woman and her family during the childbearing process. The midwife can enable the woman to have a physically rewarding and psychologically satisfying experience through sensitive and appropriate use of skills and resources. The midwife can offer a broad, in-depth insight into the rituals, practices and options surrounding childbearing within the realms of safety and the law. The midwife's principal role is to ensure the safety and wellbeing of both mother and infant. She also has the ability to inform clients and develop parenting skills within the family environment.

A client's perception of quality care occurs when the care given is sensitive and appropriate to the mother's individual needs and environment. A woman needs to have a measure of control and needs to share in the decision-making process during her care. It has to be recognized, however, that the midwife is expert in the field and has a fund of knowledge and experience on which to draw. A wise client will use this expertise to the full. A wise midwife will encourage open, honest discussion of each situation and will also admit when and if she needs to seek further advice or information before giving the client a full response. It is important that a midwife recognizes her or his skills and limitations and maintains an up-to-date knowledge of practice and of research.

A midwife needs a sound understanding of both the physical and psychological changes which take place during the childbearing process in order to be able to offer the appropriate care. Keeping up-to-date with research issues is important, but it is also important to remember that not all research is well-founded or appropriate and the ability to appraise issues critically is fundamental to the role of the midwife. It is important to assess the relevance of issues to the environment in which a midwife works and to the types of clients who may be cared for. The social norms will vary from area to area and, consequently, will influence women's choices during childbearing. A midwife needs to keep abreast of cultural, social and psychological issues in order to offer care matched to individual needs.

A clear understanding of the psychological changes during childbearing should minimize stress for the mother, since the midwife can explain the normal and discuss issues which vary from the normal and refer the client if appropriate. This can help bring about an improved professional relationship between client and carer. A sound knowledge of the pressures which a new mother undergoes should enable the midwife to offer support and encouragement as the mother learns and develops new skills of parenting. The infant also offers a challenge to the understanding of how the new infant interacts with its environment and influences that environment in a profound way. A woman who has learnt to enjoy parenting is usually a grandmother!

Clients also need to be aware that a midwife has to work within certain constraints, such as local policies, and if these are felt to be inappropriate for her care, the issue should be put to the local Supervisor of Midwives for discussion and review.

Midwifery is a demanding, challenging role. Midwives are managers, teachers, advisors and supporters as well as carers of women and families during a life crisis. Midwives must recognize not only the psychological effect that they can have on a woman and her family, but also how the midwife can influence and enhance care. The midwife needs to be aware of the effect that any one client can have on a midwife, in terms of the psychological and physical demands that a client may make, and how a midwife can cope with the stressors. Midwives need to look after their own psychological wellbeing, together with that of their colleagues. By working together in a supportive and mutually satisfying reciprocal relationship, midwives can offer a fulfilling experience for women and families in their care.

Glossary

antecedent	a happening before an event, not necessarily the cause of the event
anxiety	a state of psychological stress
attitude	a set of notions held by an individual
babbling	a baby's attempt at speech
behaviour	physical actions of an individual
bonding	a close emotional tie
communication	the process of giving, receiving, interpreting and understanding information
deprivation	withdrawal of
idiographic	an approach which looks at individuals to identify commonalities
nomothetic	an approach which looks at general principles
parenting	providing the physical, psychological, social, cultural and spiritual needs for one's young
perception	one's understanding of an event
personality	relatively enduring characteristics of an individual
pleasure principle	the purpose of the Id – to seek pleasure
privation	having no experience of

role	the part an individual plays in a social situation
self	an individual's sense of being
self-concept	how an individual views himself or herself
self-esteem	an individual's sense of worth
self-image	an individual's perception of how they appear to others
sibling	brother or sister
sibling rivalry	friction which arises between brothers or sisters
social norms	the acceptable behaviour or practices within a social group
stress	the psychological effect of an unpleasant stimulus
stressor	the cause of stress, a stimulus which may be positive or negative

References and Further Reading

Ainsworth, M.D.S., Bell, S.M.V., Stayton, D.J. (1971). 'Individual differences in strange situation behaviour of one-year-olds'. In: Schaffer, H.R. (Ed). *The Origins of Human Social Relations*. New York: Academic Press.

Ainsworth, M.D.S., Blehar, M.C., Waters, E., Wall, S. (1978). *Patterns of Attachment: A Psychological Study of the Strange Situation*. New Jersey: Lawrence Erlbaum Associates.

Allport, G.W. (1955). *Becoming – Basic Considerations for a Psychology of Personality*. Connecticut: Yale University Press.

Allport, G.W. (1961). *Pattern and Growth in Personality*. New York: Rinehart Winston.

Argyle, M. (1969). *Social Interaction*. London: Methuen.

Atkinson, R.L., Atkinson, R.C., Smith, E.E., Hilgard, E.R. (1985). *Introduction to Psychology*. 9th edn. London: Harcourt Brace Jovanovich.

Baron, R.A., Byrne, D. (1991). *Social Psychology – Understanding Human Interaction*. 6th edn. London: Allyn and Bacon.

Bowlby, J. (1969). *Attachment and Loss*. Vol. 1, Attachment. Harmondsworth: Penguin.

Bowlby, J. (1969). *Attachment and Loss*. Vol. 2, Separation. Harmondsworth: Penguin.

Bowlby, J. (1984). *Attachment and Loss*. Vol. 1, Attachment (2nd edn). Harmondsworth: Penguin Books.

Bowlby, J. (1984). *Attachment and Loss*. Vol. 1, Attachment (2nd edn). Harmondsworth: Penguin Books.

Brazelton, T.B. (1976). 'Early parent-infant reciprocity'. In: Vaughan, V.C., Brazelton, T.B. (Eds). *The Family: Can it be Saved?* Chicago: Yearbook Medical Publishers.

Burnard, P. (1991). *Coping with Stress in the Health Professions*. London: Chapman and Hall.

Cooper, C.S., Dunst, C.J., Vance, S.D. (1990). 'The effect of social support on adolescent mothers' styles of parent-child interaction as measured on three separate occasions'. *Adolescence*, Vol. XXV, No. 97, Spring.

Darwin, C. (1872). *The Expression of the Emotions in Man and Animals*. London: Philosophical Library.

de Selincourt, K. (1991). 'Dignified in death... babies born before 28 weeks gestation'. *Nursing Times*, 87(29), pp. 16–17.

Department of Health (1993). *Changing Childbirth*, Parts 1 and 11, London: HMSO.

Dunn, J. (1988). *The Beginnings of Social Understanding*. Oxford: Blackwell

Elster, A.B., McAnarney, E.R., Lamb, M.E. (1983). 'Parental behaviour of adolescent mothers'. *Pediatrics*, 71, pp.494–503.

Eysenck, H.J. (1976). *The Measurement of Personality*. Baltimore: Baltimore University Park Press.

Eysenck, H.J., Eysenck, S.B.G. (1969). *Personality Structure and Measurement*. London: Routledge and Kegan Paul.

Fantz, R. (1961). *Scientific American*, 204, pp. 66–72.

Flint, C. (1986). *Sensitive Midwifery*. Oxford: Heinemann.

Gieve, K. (1989). *Balancing Acts – On Being a Mother*. London: Virago.

Goring, R. (1992). *Dictionary of Beliefs and Religion*. Edinburgh: Chambers.

Gross, R.D. (1992). *Psychology: The Science of Mind and Behaviour*. London: Hodder and Stoughton.

Hershenson, M. (1967). 'Development of the perception of form'. *Psychological Bulletin*, Vol. 67, pp. 326–36.

Hinton, J. (1975). *Dying*. Harmondsworth: Penguin Books.

Jenkins, R. (1995). *The Law and the Midwife*. Oxford: Blackwell.

Kohner, N., Henley, A. (1991). *Miscarriage, Stillbirth and Neonatal Death; Guidelines for Professionals*. London: SANDS.

Kohner, N., Henley, A. (1991). *When a Baby Dies*. London: SANDS

Kubler-Ross, E. (1978). *On Death and Dying*. London: Tavistock Publications.

Lorenz, K.Z. (1935). 'The companion in the bird's world'. *Auk*, 54, pp. 245–73.

Moss, H.A. (1967). 'Sex, age and state as determinants of mother-infant interaction'. *Merrill-Palmer Quarterly*, 13, pp. 19–36. (Mothers' contacts with infant boys and girls)

Murray-Parkes, C. (1986). *Bereavement: Studies of Grief in Adult Life*. 2nd edn. London: Tavistock Publications.

Niven, N. (1994). *Health Psychology*. 2nd edition, London: Churchill Livingstone.

Oakley, A. (1980). *Women Confined: Towards a Sociology of Childbirth*. Oxford: Martin Robertson.

Onions, C.T. (1973). *The Shorter Oxford English Dictionary*. Oxford: Clarendon Press.

Parkes, C.M. (1985). *Bereavement: Studies of Grief in Adult Life*. 2nd edn. Harmondsworth: Penguin Books.

Parkes, C.M., Weiss, R.S. (1983). *Recovery from Bereavement*. New York: Basic Books.

Plath, S. (1990). 'Metaphors'. In: *Collected Poems*. London: Faber and Faber.

Postle, D. (1988). *The Mind Gymnasium*. London: Macmillan.

Price, J. (1988). *Motherhood – What It Does To Your Mind*. London: Pandora.

Prince, J., Adams, M. (1987). *The Psychology of Childbirth*. London: Churchill Livingstone.

Reber, A.S. (1985). *Dictionary of Psychology*. Harmondsworth: Penguin.

Royal College of Midwives/Health Education Council Report (1985). *Midwives and Stillbirth*. London: RCM.

Rutter, M. (1981). *Maternal Deprivation Reassessed*. 2nd edn. Harmondsworth: Penguin.

Schaffer, R. (1971). *The Growth of Sociability*. London: Fontana.

Schaffer, R. (1977). *Mothering*. London: Fontana.

Spear, P.D., Penrod, S.D., Baker, T.B. (1988). *Psychology: Perspectives on Behaviour*. Chichester: John Wiley and Sons.

Stern, D.N. (1977). *The First Relationship: Infant and Mother*. London: Fontana.

Stratton, D.N. (1982). 'Rhythmic functions in the newborn'. *The Psychobiology of the Human Newborn*. New York: Wiley.

Stratton, P., Hayes, N. (1993). *A Student's Dictionary of Psychology*. 2nd edn. London: Edward Arnold.

UKCC (1993). *Midwives Rules*. London: United Kingdom Central Council for Nursing, Midwifery and Health Visiting.

Wiemann, J.M. (1985). 'Interpersonal control and regulations in conversation'. In: Street, R.L., Cappella, J.N. (Eds). *Sequence and Pattern in Communicative Behaviour*. London: Edward Arnold.

Winnicott, D.W. (1964). *The Child, The Family and the Outside World*. London: Pelican.

Wolff, P.H. (1969). 'The natural history of crying and other vocalisations in early infancy'. In: Foss, B.M. (Ed). *Determinants of Infant Behaviour*. Vol. 4, London: Methuen.

Index